STRANGERS
IN OUR *Home*

An Introspective View Of Caregivers
From A Registered Nurse's Point Of View

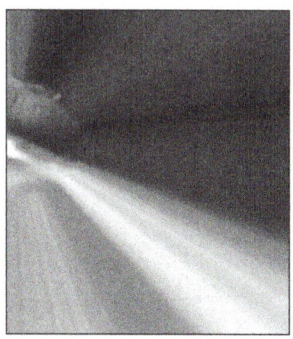

CHERYL BROWN

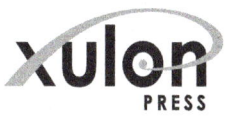

Copyright © 2015 by CHERYL BROWN

STRANGERS IN MY HOME
*An Introspective View Of Caregivers From A Registered Nurse's Point Of View*by
CHERYL BROWN

Printed in the United States of America.

ISBN 9781498466073

All rights reserved solely by the author. The author guarantees all contents are original and do not infringe upon the legal rights of any other person or work. No part of this book may be reproduced in any form without the permission of the author. The views expressed in this book are not necessarily those of the publisher.

Unless otherwise indicated, Scripture quotations taken from the King James Version (KJV) – *public domain.*

www.xulonpress.com

ACKNOWLEDGEMENTS

I would like to acknowledge the staff at the Washington D.C. VAMC for their support in providing caregivers to my husband and placing us into the Community Based Veterans Home Program.

Special acknowledgement to the Paralyzed Veterans of America for providing an opportunity to co-author an article as it related to getting Caregivers in the home.

A very special acknowledgement for my husband James. He gives me all I need to remain fulfilled, balanced and true to myself. Without him, the first 2 books would not have been possible. They are the creation of our years of labor and love together.

Caregiving is a labor of love.

"Be shepherds of God's flock that is under your care, serving as overseers—not because you must, but because you are willing, as God wants you to be; not greedy for money, but eager to serve; not lording it over those entrusted to you, but being examples to the flock. And when the Chief Shepherd appears, you will receive the crown of glory that will never fade away." —1 Peter 5:2–4

Chapter One

THE LIAR

In our first book, *I Want to Dance with my Wife Again,* my husband and I chronicle our challenges of living with a diagnosis of Multiple Sclerosis (MS).

It was exactly twenty-six years and four months ago that James was given a diagnosis of Multiple Sclerosis. We had dated for 2 years before getting married by a Justice of the Peace in Virginia Beach, Virginia. I was not so sure that I wanted to remarry since I had been married before. It did not work out, we were too young and from different worlds.

My first husband saw the world in colors through his smoke hazed marijuana glasses and I saw it in black and white. We were like oil and water. Our union was not a good one. I vowed to never marry again.

A few years later, James steps into my life. He was the visual of everything that I wanted in a husband. He loved and supported his children. He respected women as evidenced by his love for his grandmother, mother and sisters. He went to church and he even believed in God.

We agreed early in our relationship that God would always be first in our life.

He had joined the United States Marine Corps when he graduated from high school in 1972.

One year later, he was honorably and medically discharged from the Marine Corps because he was told by one of the physicians at the Portsmouth Naval Hospital that his "immune system was messed up".

James told me that while he was stationed at Camp Le June in South Carolina, he and his platoon were moved out of their barracks and made to sleep in Quonset Huts set up outside the barracks.

Years later, the Marine Corps admits there were problems with the well water. There was a Dry Cleaning company that dumped dry cleaning solvents in the well water. Subsequently, many Marines and their family members developed neurological diseases or symptoms which they have been compensated for.

It took thirty years to find evidence that something happened to my husband when he was in the Marine Corps. It took that long to start receiving some compensation and assistance for medical care. It took thirteen years into our marriage to receive some relief.

After I graduated from Norfolk State University's Nursing Program in May of 1986, I needed a reliable car to get to and from work. It was during that time, nurses worked multiple shifts. Whatever your supervisor assigned, you worked it. Days, evenings, nights or weekends.

The Liar

There was no complaining or crying to your supervisor's boss because you got a schedule you did not like. You just dealt with it. It built character.

After going to several car dealerships in the Norfolk-Portsmouth area, I was told that I needed a co-signer for a car. I called my Great Uncle Buddy to help me with my dilemma.

When I called, his wife, Aunt Bert answered the phone.

"Hello, Aunt Bert, How are you doing?"

"Who's this, Cheryl?"

"Yes, ma'am."

"You want to talk to your Uncle Buddy?"

"Yes ma'am."

"He's not home right now, what do you want me to tell him?"

"Aunt Bert, I have been going to different car dealerships to try to buy a reliable car so that I can get to and from work without problems and haven't been able to get one because they tell me that I need a co-signer on my car loan. I was calling to see if Uncle Buddy would do that for me."

"Well, Cheryl, you know my grandson James sells cars and…he just walked in the door."

I can hear her talking to her grandson and handing him the phone.

"Hello?"

"Hi."

"Who's this?"

"This is Cheryl, Buddy's niece. Your cousin."

"You might be Buddy's niece, but you are not my cousin."

"What do you mean?"

"Buddy is not my grandfather, he is the only grandfather that I have ever known, but George Brown is my grandfather. Grandma and Buddy did not have any children."

"Oh. I didn't know that. Uncle Buddy moved away from the Eastern Shore of Virginia long before I was born and I only saw him on special occasions. He was always the Hero and was treated as such when he visited. Now that we have that out of the way, I called to ask Uncle Buddy to co-sign a loan for me so that I can get a more reliable car."

"You know I sell cars."

"Yes, your grandmother told me."

"I can get you in a car."

"Really?"

"Yes. What kind of work do you do?"

"I am a Nurse."

"What kind of Nurse?"

I am really not liking this guy. The last time I saw him at church, he had a Geri Curl hanging on his shoulder and a gold tooth in the front. His hands were softer and better looking than mine. Can someone say "Player, Player?"

"I am a Registered Nurse. Does that help?"

"Yes."

From there, he asked the usual questions, what is your salary, how long have you worked at your current job, etc.

The very next day, I got a phone call from Mr. Salesman Extraordinaire. He told me that he had a car for me and that I did not need a co-signer.

Yeah! I guess he really does know his stuff. A few days later, he brought the car by my apartment for me to test drive!

I was super excited!

The next day, he picked me up and took me to the dealership to sign the paperwork for my new car. It was a repossession. He said that the girl who had the car before me had brought it fraudulently by using her mother's checks. All she did was drive the car and never made a payment on it.

It was beautiful. It was gold in color with black interior. A Dodge Daytona.

We started dating a few months after that.

Two years later we were married.

Twenty-six years later we are writing our second book.

In this book, I want my readers to understand the frustrations that we have experienced in trying to find caregivers to assist with caring for my husband while in the home. I have heard lots of horror stories as it related to situations similar to ours, but have not seen books written about it.

I hope that this book will set the groundwork to develop nursing programs that will weed out those who are incompetent or do not have the heart to care for others.

Twenty years after my husband's diagnosis of Multiple Sclerosis, he started requiring more assistance with daily activities. I still worked and could not afford to stay home and contacted the Veteran's Administration in Washington, D.C.

The Coordinator of the program contacted one of their contracted agencies who provided us ten hours of care per week.

The person sent to work with my husband was named Terri.

Terri seemed to be a nice person by all accounts. She was in her thirties, had a ten-year-old son and was unmarried. She lived in La Plata, Maryland which was only a few miles from where we lived. Terri was about 5 feet tall and slight in size. She was friendly and talkative.

On her first day, I stayed home to help her around the house. James was ever watchful and distrustful. It was a beautiful summer day. The sun was shining and the birds were singing. Our neighborhood was very quiet because most people were at work.

My boss at Paralyzed Veterans had given me the day off to help get our Nursing Assistant settled in at home with James. My husband did not want any parts of this and was not so sure he wanted a stranger in our home.

"James, you know that I have to work and hopefully, this person will work out so that I can continue working outside the home to help with paying the bills."

"Yeah, I know. But I have Chi."

Chi-Square Brown is our six-year-old German Shepherd. James trained her to pick up bottles or anything he dropped on the floor. She fetched the newspaper for him from the driveway.

One day when Chi went out to get the paper, the trash truck had arrived and the guys were collecting the trash. Chi, ran to one of the men with the newspaper in her mouth to give it to him and James said the man ran down the street screaming. He had to call Chi back to the house and she happily brought the paper to him.

He apologized to the crew and told them that Chi only wanted to give him the paper.

They laughed and went on their way.

"I know that Chi can pick up bottles that you drop on the floor, but she can't help you in the bathroom."

"It is hard for me to try to work knowing that you are having problems getting around in the house."

"I know that, but I am not so sure this is going to work."

"Let's give it a try."

Terry was due at Nine O'clock. She was scheduled to work from 9 A.M. to 12 Noon three days a week. Mondays, Wednesdays, and Fridays.

"Good Morning."

"Hi. My name is Terri."

"Hi, Terri, my name is Cheryl. This is James and our dog's name is Chi."

"Oh! I didn't know that you had a dog."

"Are you afraid of dogs? Chi is well behaved."

"No, I'm not. Will I have to do anything with her?"

"No, she is paper-trained. She uses the bathroom in the garage. I put the paper down on top of plastic trash bags and clean it up when I come home."

"Oh. Okay, then. I'm okay with that."

"Come on in. Chi, go sit on you bed." Chi walks over to her bed by the sofa in the Family Room and lies down.

"James, this is Terri. Terri this is my husband James."

"Good morning, Mr. James."

"Good morning."

"Do you want me to call you Mr. James or Mr. Brown?"

"Mr. James is okay."

"James, I am going to show Terry around and let her know how she can help you around the house."

"Terri, James is pretty independent, his biggest problem is falling. He is starting to fall a little more. He has Multiple

Sclerosis and with this disease, losing balance is one of the biggest problems."

"Is that a muscle disease?"

"It's a disease of the nerves which eventually affects the muscles."

"I think that I have taken care of someone who had that."

"Okay. Here is the bathroom where he will come when he has to go. He may require some assistance with getting on and off the commode. Just stay close if he needs help he will let you know."

"He may want to go upstairs, and we will need you to help him upstairs. We don't have a chair lift yet. Hopefully, it will come soon."

"Sometimes he might want to go outside with the dog and play with her. He has a scooter in the garage and may need some help down the steps to the scooter so that he can go outside."

"Does he go outside often?"

"Not too often. If he wants to go out, he will let you know."

Just before it was time for Terri to leave, I gave her our emergency contact information.

"Is this something you think that you will like?"

"Yes, I think so, but I need to work more hours."

"Okay. We certainly need someone more than the VA is giving us now. Let me see what I can do."

A few days later, I informed Terri that I had worked out a deal with her agency to have her work an additional 5 hours with James. She was happy about that.

The Liar

Soon after that, James made me aware that Terri had been late to work or not coming at all.

I called the agency to speak to the nursing supervisor.

"Hello. May I speak to the nursing supervisor?"

"Okay. Hold one moment."

"Hello, this is the nursing supervisor."

"Yes. My name is Cheryl Brown and my husband, James is a client of yours. What is your name?"

"My name is Paul."

"Paul, I'm calling to talk to you about one of your Nursing Assistants by the name of Terri."

"Terri. Oh yes!"

"How is Terri when it comes to responsibility? Is she usually on time? Does she report to work as scheduled?'

"Well, we have found with Terri, that we have to make her write everything down to make sure we are on the same page."

"Oh really?"

"Well, she has been missing days of work and tells my husband that she called you to let you know that she wouldn't be in."

"She called us to tell us she was not needed at your home."

"Okay. I see what's going on. She's playing it from both ends."

"I tell you what. See if you can find us someone else."

"Mrs. Brown, we can talk to her. It's hard for us to find people to cover the area you live in."

"It seems that a problem has already been identified and I don't see how it's going to get better. She's a liar."

"Mrs. Brown, let me see what I can do. If we can talk to Terri and tell her that this is her last chance, would you be willing to let her come?"

"Can you hold one moment?"

"James. Are you willing to let Terri come back if the agency talks to her?"

"I don't really need her here. She just lies so much."

"Okay."

"Paul? James says he doesn't want to chance it. If you can find someone else, that would be great."

Fortunately or unfortunately for us, we were not able to find anyone else to come work for us from that agency.

James also told me of other situations with this particular Nursing Assistant that I was not aware of. One day, her car broke down in the driveway. She called someone to pick her up and then had someone come back to our home to work on her car to get it started.

I think that she wanted us to pay the guy for fixing her car.

We didn't and after that her coming to work was not a guarantee.

We called the VA and requested another agency.

We got what we asked for. Sometimes you do have to be careful what you ask for. You just really might get it.

Chapter 2

BAIT AND SWITCH

After Terri, James was not so sure he wanted anyone else to come into our home to work with him. He was becoming more and more unstable. I still had to work to make ends meet. His VA pension was not enough to cover even the mortgage.

I called the VA Home Care Coordinator to ask for another agency.

"Hello. May I speak to Drucilla Davis?"

"This is Drucilla Davis. How may I help you?"

"Drucilla. This is Cheryl Brown, I'm calling on behalf of my husband, James. We would like to try another nursing agency. The one we were with could not find anyone to work with us. Do you know of another agency in our area that can help us?"

"Okay. I know of one right there in Fort Washington, Maryland that can help you."

"I'll give them a call to see if they can help you."

"Okay. Thank you."

A few days later we received a call from the nursing agency in Fort Washington, Maryland. The coordinator, a Registered Nurse came out to do the assessment.

She and I hit it off immediately. We knew some of the same people. We were both belonged to the African Methodist Episcopal Church (A.M.E.). This had to work, right?

She and I talked about how she got the nursing assistants for her company and about the nursing sorority she was in.

Another clue. Recruitment for the sorority.

The first Nursing Assistant sent to help my husband was fairly young, but mature for her age. She was very competent and we thought that we had hit the jackpot until, we got that fatal phone call from the agency a few months later.

"Hello. Cheryl?"

"Yes?"

"This is Regina from the nursing agency. I was calling to let you know that your Nursing Assistant will not be coming back."

"Why?"

"Her husband was seriously ill and just died."

"What?"

"She has to make funeral preparations and the family is from Nigeria, Africa."

"Oh. How sad. She was very competent and good."

"I know, she was actually a Licensed Practical Nurse and wanted to work to keep up her skills."

"I knew there was something different about her."

"I will look around at my staff and send someone to help your husband out."

"Okay. Thank you."

A few days later, Regina called to let me know that she had another Nursing Assistant by the name of Sherri. She lived in Accokeek and had been working with the agency for quite some time.

When Sherri arrived. I gave her the tour and spiel. James was not enthused in the least bit.

Sherri settled in okay and was always willing to do whatever I asked. She agreed to babysit with extra payment.

I thought all was well until I noticed that the chair arm on my newly purchased sofa was unraveling. It looked as though someone was pulling the fabric from the chair.

One Sunday when I was in the kitchen cooking, it started getting a little warm. I went to the thermostat to adjust it to a cooler temperature. When it wouldn't work and I pulled the cover off, Amiaya who was three at the time started stomping her foot on the floor.

"Mommy. Miss Sherri had that on the floor and she put her foot on it and did, ump, ump, ump with her feet."

"What were you doing when she did this?"

"She told me to turn my head around and not look, but I looked anyway."

"Why didn't you tell me?"

"I don't know."

"Mommy are you going to call the police and put Miss Sherri in jail?"

"Do you think that she should go to jail?"

"Yes."

"I am going to call the agency and tell them not to send her back out again."

Over the next couple of months, the agency sent a couple more girls out to help with my husband. They were very young. Inexperienced. Looking for work.

One girl had to be dropped off and picked up by her boyfriend every time she came to work. This made James very uneasy.

Another girl only sat on the sofa in front of the big screened Television and watched T.V.

Instead of going upstairs to check on James. She would stand at the bottom of the stairs and call up, "James are you okay."

One day, James called me while I was at work to let me know that he had been stuck in the bathroom for over one and one half hours without anyone coming to check on him.

I called the agency and told them that my husband needed assistance and the Nursing Assistant was sitting downstairs watching T.V.

The agency called her to let her know that she needed to go check on my husband.

She lasted a few more days.

When I threatened to leave this agency, they sent their special operations person to help with our situation.

When Raydean showed up. I was at my wit's end. Amiaya was running around the house and James was sitting in the family room watching the T.V.

I was starting to wonder what have I gotten myself into? A three-year-old, a disabled husband, a full-time job and a whole lot of other responsibilities.

What was I really thinking to take a child into our home and raise her with my husband's assistance? His health was steadily deteriorating. He needed care.

I talked to Raydean and she went into the family room to talk to James.

She drove up in a Mercedes.

She had to have her ducks in a row didn't she?

She seemed mature, clean, experienced.

She had to be the one, right?

Raydean started work the next week.

She agreed to take Amiaya to KinderCare for me so that I could get to work a little earlier.

I would dress, wash Amiaya's face and brush her teeth before I went to work so that all Raydean had to do was take her to school.

I paid her fifty dollars a week to do this for us.

It worked for 2 months until Raydean told my husband that she was going to work for a Nursing Home so that she could get more hours and benefits.

The week before she left us, she claimed that she had a heart attack and did not know it until a doctor's visit.

After Raydean left, we called to cancel with the agency. The owner made us aware that we would have to pay them extra money for the hours that Raydean had worked because the VA would only pay for a restricted number of hours.

Little did I know that my husband was becoming distressed and depressed?

Chapter 3

THE OTHER AGENCY

When I contacted Mrs. Davis at the VA to let her know the course of events. She told me that there was one more agency that she could refer me to and this agency was tops.

We waited to hear from this agency based in Bethesda, not far from where I worked.

I made the agency owner aware of the previous problems that I had encountered before and that I needed to work to complete a project that I was involved in at Walter Reed National Military Medical Center.

They assured me that they had the staff to meet our needs.

Mary was very neat and washed all of the time, but decided to leave after taking my husband to physical therapy appointments at National Rehabilitation hospital.

She recruited one of her friends to work with James. A male.

This guy did not bathe himself well at all. James would not let him assist him with any personal care needs.

His body odor was ingrained in our family room sofa. I had to remove the covers from the pillows and wash them.

I called the agency to ask for someone else.

They sent another one of their top Nursing Assistants to work with us. I do not know her name because she did not last one day.

My husband had an accident and could not get to the bathroom in a timely fashion. This Nursing Assistant had to help him change into clean clothing.

When Amiaya and I got home, the house reeked of bodily fluids. I had to help my dear husband upstairs to shower and then clean the sofa cushions and shampoo the carpet in the family room.

In addition to that, I still had to cook supper and help our daughter with her homework. Thank God she was just in Kindergarten.

I called the agency to report to them what had happened on the way to work.

They refused to work with me and dropped us.

They labeled us as difficult.

Chapter 4

VETERANS HOME BASED COMMUNITY PROGRAM

After we were dropped from the agency, I called our nurse practitioner, Cathy Denobile and Drucilla Davis, the VA Home Care Coordinator again to see if they had any more recommendations/suggestions for us.

We needed help.

I was not finished with the Level 2 Trauma Center Verification at Bethesda.

The contract employees working for me were making my life more and more difficult, trying to make me look incompetent in the eyes of my superiors. They were not capable of doing the job themselves and did not understand what needed to be done. They did not have the negotiation skills or competence to make it happen.

The first contract employee, Kathy Curry was in the position of Trauma Program Manager before Walter Reed Army Medical Center merged with Bethesda Naval Hospital to become Walter Reed National Military Medical Center. I was a Graduated Scale (GS) employee. Contract employees by Federal Law were not allowed to supervise GS employees.

Ms. Curry was not made aware of this fact before the merger. We had been the best of friends and were on the best of terms before I moved into my office which was down the hall from her.

It soon became evident that Ms. Curry was into the glamour of the position. She knew all of the Wounded Warriors by name and made sure everyone knew it. She sent news clippings or articles out to everyone when they were available.

She did not have a clue about how to make this program stand up to become a Trauma Center.

My experience from the old Walter Reed Army Medical Center had given me the edge on her. I organized a Consultation Site Visit with the American College of Surgeons under the guidance of Colonel Stephen Flaherty.

The site visit was very successful. The surveyors only found thirteen discrepancies with our facility even though we were in the process of a merger.

It was my job as the Trauma Program Manager to ensure that all of the electronic records kept on the Wounded Warriors were transferred to Bethesda without compromise. The records were highly sensitive and contained classified information as it related to the locations of the soldiers when they were injured.

These efforts to ensure swift transfer of those records involved every one of my staff members who had responsibilities to ensure this transfer happened with zero deficits. One week before the actual merger, my staff stopped abstracting the medical records.

Veterans Home Based Community Program

Even though these efforts had stopped, we were required to meet every week on a Thursday to discuss these soldiers and their injuries in an international Teleconference. The teleconferences included persons from the Secretary of the Army down to the nurses, surgeons, technicians who cared for the Wounded Warriors from the field to the Station Hospitals.

During the merger, I scheduled appointments with the Information Technology (IT) personnel to ensure our program was able to meet their DICAP standards for migration and would not be erased from the network which would hinder our efforts to continue to abstract information from the medical records.

Coordinated efforts were put in place with the personnel in San Antonio Texas at the Institute of Surgical Research (ISR). The director of their program, Sheralyn Wright and I worked closely to ensure this process was successful. We could not lose this information.

Mrs. Curry had told me that this process was not going to work because she had met with the head of the Information Technology department and was told that we would only be able to hook the computers up in one room and work on a router to abstract and share the data.

She tried to hinder all efforts to make this one of many processes fail. She had also lost the installation disk from the Institute of Surgical Research that she had originally been given before our arrival to install the software for the Department of Defense Trauma Registry (DODTR).

Her cohort, Mrs. Fluerette Etienne was just as culpable. She was hired into the position of Performance Improvement (PI) Coordinator for the program.

The PI Coordinator was responsible for ensuring that all of the data collected on the Wounded Warriors was reliable and reproducible. This person was also responsible for collecting the statistics to place into the Pre Review Questionnaire for the American College of Surgeons prior to their visit.

After a few weeks, it became obvious to me and my staff that we were encountering counter measures to make this program unsuccessful because Mrs. Curry and Mrs. Etienne were not used to having appropriate supervision and held accountable for their job descriptions.

They never reported to me or requested time off in an appropriate manner. They would report to my supervisor because they had a working relationship with him and he would approve whatever they wanted. He never sent them back to me for approval. I would find out they were going to be absent on the day of.

One day, Mrs. Etienne, who was a Captain in the Naval Reserves made arrangements to dress in uniform and go to meet her nurses at Andrews Air Force Base as they arrived from their deployment in Afghanistan.

This should have never happened. She could not separate her Reserve responsibilities from her work responsibilities. She was ordered by another one of my supervisors that she would not be able to come to her office during her reserve duty, but report to her work area only. She tried to get paid for working during her reserve duty tour.

It took over one and one half years to get them out of their positions and have someone finally assist me in finding qualified individuals to work to make the program successful.

In September, 2013, the physicians from the American College of Surgeons visited our facility and we were awarded the Level 2 Trauma Center Verification. My staff and I who had worked so hard since 2009 to achieve this status were not mentioned in any of the nationally publicized news articles. Only in the local hospital newsletter.

By this time, I was so exhausted. I was continually ill with colds and the Flu. I called out sick at least every other week.

I applied for a lesser position at Fort Belvoir as a Case Manager and left that position after four weeks due to exhaustion.

My husband had been awarded a lump sum award from the Veterans Administration in June of 2013 which made it easy for me to make the decision to leave my Federal job to care for myself, him and our daughter.

Cathy referred us to the Baltimore VA for their home-based program.

We were then contacted by Mrs. Joanne Carnathan, the coordinator at the Prince George's County Department on Aging. She came to our home and evaluated my husband for the highest tier of care.

We were awarded 40 hours of care per week. Paid for by the VA.

We were happy.

Who would we call?

Raydean, of course!

She and Mary were the two best Nursing Assistants we had worked with. James was hesitant about her, because he stated that she walked out on us, and he did not want her back.

"Cheryl, she abandoned me and said she was going to work at a nursing home for the insurance. When someone does that, you don't invite them back," said James.

"James, we need help. Was she that bad of a nursing assistant?" I responded.

"No."

"Could you work with her until I finish the verification at my job?" I asked.

"I really want you to stay home and work with me. I know that I can get better if you do that," James professed.

"James, you know that I have to finish what I started in the name of God, country and the military members. This can help us in the long run, and it is groundbreaking work for the hospital."

"James, you know that I have been a nurse since I was eighteen years old."

"I Know."

"I started out as a Licensed Practical Nurse (LPN) and went on to graduate from Norfolk State University in 1983 with my Associate's Degree in Nursing. Then I went back to get my Bachelor's Degree from Norfolk State and my Masters in Public Health from Eastern Virginia Medical School."

"Cheryl, I know that."

"You also know that I have had many experiences in my nursing career, but this one position incorporates all of my talents and skills in nursing to achieve this award for the hospital.

As I near the end of my working career, this will be a crowning achievement."

"You don't have to work; we can afford for you to stay home now. God answered my prayers and made it so."

"Please let me call Raydean and see if she will work until I finish this project next year at least?" I asked.

"If you would stay home with me, I just know that I can get better. I don't want her coming back to our home."

"James, I know that you love me, but don't you think that is a little selfish? I love what I do. I am going to call Raydean, unless you have someone else you know that we can call on short notice."

"No. I don't."

"Hello. Raydean? This is Cheryl Brown, James Brown's wife. You worked for us for a short period of time. James said you were a good Aide. Would you be willing to come work with us with a new program through the VA?" I asked.

We were not sure, she still had the same phone number since the call went to voicemail.

One week later, she called.

I called Mrs. Carnathan to make her aware of the person who was coming to help us and wanted to know what needed to be done.

We scheduled to have the accountant meet with us at home so that Raydean could complete the paperwork.

I left work early.

James had been moved to the downstairs office which was now his bedroom.

While I was talking to Mrs. Carnathan and the Accountant, Raydean went in to talk to James.

All was set.

That evening, James told me that Raydean had come in to talk to him and told him.

"Hey, Mr. Brown, how are you doing?"

"I'm okay."

"You know since I left you and Mrs. Brown, my husband lost his job and almost lost his life."

"How so?"

"He became sick and had to go to the hospital. He had a ruptured appendix and almost died from it. He did not have sick leave and since he was out of work for so long, he could not go back to his job."

"Wow."

"I lost my job because I was at his bedside 24/7 because I know how hospitals are."

"That must have been hard."

"We lost our house. Kenneth lost his truck. We are living in 2 separate places. He lives with his sister. Me and our daughter live with my brother."

I was so happy to have someone that we had worked with before who could assist with care of my husband. I did not heed the warning signs or tone of the conversation James had relayed to me.

I did not know the story she was laying on my husband before she even started working. I did not know she was setting us up to get all we had.

"Raydean. Come here for a moment."

"Is fifteen dollars an hour okay?"

"Yes it is. When can I start?"

Mrs. Carnathan, when can she start?

"Well you have to start on the 1st or the 15th. Since the 1st has already passed, you will start on the 15th."

"Okay. We will see you on the 15th."

"So, Mrs. Brown, you know her?"

"Yes. She used to work for us before and James really liked her."

"It's good when things work out."

"Yes it is."

Things went well in the beginning. Raydean settled in and James seemed to be doing okay and in a good mood when Amiaya and I got home.

A few months into this deal, Raydean started changing a little. It seemed that every chance she got, she talked about money.

There was always something wrong with her car. She needed to get an apartment. She and her family were planning a family vacation in Ocean City for the weekend.

Now mind you, we were giving her an additional fifty dollars a week for taking Amiaya to KinderCare and then school.

Whenever, we were out of town and she was scheduled to work, we paid her out of pocket. She always got the holidays off because the VA only paid for a total of 160 hours per month and when there were extra days worked in the month, we compensated by giving the day off or paying out of pocket.

She was making money hand over fist.

One day when I was home, I heard Raydean going through my kitchen cabinets. When I came downstairs and asked if she was preparing food for James, she said:

"Mrs. Brown, I was looking through your cabinets to see where things were in the event Mr. Brown wanted to have me cook for him."

This is the woman who said she would do anything but cook.

"Oh really?"

"Yes, those pans you have are they American Homes?"

"Yes. I bought them when I was in college over thirty years ago on a payment plan."

"Those are very nice and they last a long time. I especially like those cast iron skillets you have too."

"Yes, those came from my husband's great uncle and have been in the family a long time."

When a woman starts snooping through your things that is not a good sign. There is an immediate disregard for the Lady of the House because it seemed as though since she was taking care of my husband, she deserved the same things I had.

I should have fired her on the spot, *but I really needed the help*.

James told me to put up security cameras in the house.

Disney DVD's suddenly appeared in Amiaya's room as well as shelves, pictures and a Disney clock.

She said she asked Mr. Brown if it was okay to put the clock up on the wall in my daughter's room.

Amiaya and I like watching Tyler Perry's Madea character. We have almost every movie he has ever made. Since the fourth of July weekend was coming up. We decided to get the DVD's out and leave them by the DVD player in the family room.

We were going to have a Madea weekend.

One evening after we got home, Amiaya went over to the TV in the family room and kept saying, "Look Mommy." She was holding one of the DVD jackets.

When I finally paid attention to her and went over to see what she was talking about, I could not find our Madea DVD's.

I searched high and low for those DVD's and could not find them.

James said that Raydean had been talking about a camping trip that she, her husband, daughter and some neighborhood kids were going on that weekend. Her husband was the father figure many of the children lacked.

A man who did not work and gave little girls candy was the father figure for the neighborhood.

I texted Raydean and told her to bring my DVD's back to our home. I also told her that she could have asked for them. She forgot that she had told us that she was going camping that weekend with her husband and some of the neighborhood children.

I felt that something else was missing, but couldn't quite put my finger on it.

When Raydean called back, she said that she did not have my DVD's.

On that Tuesday, when she returned to work, I stayed home to talk to her. She said that she had not taken my DVD's and if she wanted to borrow them, she knew to ask us for them.

"Okay. So where are the Disney DVD's that you gave to Amiaya?"

"I don't know what you are talking about, Mrs. Brown."

Oh. So now you want to play games.

"Do you still want to work here?"

"Mrs. Brown, I am not sure. I will let you know by this evening."

"Okay. I will not have people taking from me. I am way too good to you. If you need something, ask us for it."

Little did I know that she would actually take it literally?

Then it happened.

James called me at work and told me that Raydean had asked him to lend her eight hundred dollars.

I played along with the game on the phone.

We had just installed Verizon Home Monitoring Cameras in the home and I was able to watch her remotely.

I saw a lady pacing back and forth in the Family Room.

A lady on the phone with someone.

A lady who kept sitting and then getting up to walk to the room that James was in.

I did not like this.

I was not comfortable.

I called our coordinator and told her what had occurred.

I called Raydean when I got home and told her that we were letting her go because she was trying to extort money from us.

I reported her to the board of nursing.

She was told not to come by our home again.

She showed up one morning as I was taking Amiaya to school.

I almost backed the van over her while she was walking up our driveway.

I think that she considered getting hit by the van, but realized that she was not supposed to be on our property at all.

She wanted to go in and say goodbye to James.

"No. You cannot go in and say goodbye to him."

"Can you sign my time sheet for me?"

"Okay."

I signed her sheet.

She asked for a hug.

She said, "You know that you took away my livelihood?"

I said, "You know in ten months you have made over thirty thousand dollars with the perks that we have given you?"

She looked astonished.

"Your average salary working for the VA in this program is around $28,000.00 a year. I calculated by the end of the year at the rate you are going, you will have made close to $50,000.00 from working with us."

I closed the garage door and parted ways with her.

She stalked James on Facebook.

I blocked her.

After Raydean left, we advertised on Care.Com.

James and I interviewed several people and explained the program that he was in.

He chose Angel.

Angel seemed too good to be true.

I've learned that when something seems too good to be true, it usually is too good to be true.

Angel came in and sold all of her wares to us that first week. She had been a teacher in the Philippines. Her sons were honor students at University of Maryland in the Engineering program. She had a house cleaning business. She could clean our home for us and she could tutor our daughter for us.

She offered to tutor Amiaya to make sure she stayed current in school.

She offered to clean our home.

She stated that she could take care of my husband and get him back on his feet.

She was hired as a caregiver for my husband and a tutor for our daughter.

Amiaya became more confused in school requiring intervention. The teachers were beginning to wonder if she indeed spoke English.

I only allowed her to clean our home twice. She did not clean the handles on the tubs or showers. She only scrubbed the wood floor with a substance that made me nauseous.

She did not wash the rugs in the bathroom.

She did not dust the blades on the ceiling fan in my bedroom.

She broke the custom curtains in the Dining and Living Room.

She started comparing what I had in my home to what she had in hers.

I realized that this cleaning business was probably a way to clean one's house out versus cleaning it up.

I started cleaning my own home.

Walter Reed National Military Medical Center had finally become a Level 2 Trauma Center.

I looked diligently for a job closer to home at Fort Belvoir. There was one on USA jobs. I applied for the Case Manager position.

I interviewed for the position.

I was offered the position.

I transferred to Fort Belvoir, Virginia to become a Case Manager.

After four weeks, I realized that I really needed to be home with my husband to ensure he received decent nursing care.

I was paying through the nose for Angel to work overtime until we came home because James could not be left alone.

I sat down one day to calculate the amount paid to Angel for Overtime, gas to and from work, before and after care for Amiaya and miscellaneous expenses and it totaled my yearly salary.

Some days when I came from work, he had washcloths from head to toe on his body.

"Angel, why does he have so many washcloths on him?"

"I thought that he might get cold and needed to have something to keep him warm."

"He has a blanket on the foot of the bed and the thermostat can be adjusted to warm up the house."

"I don't bother with that thermostat. I don't bother other people's stuff."

Angel did not know how to do basic hygiene.

James said she would use wet ones to give him a bath.

She would do this while leaving his clothes on.

She would not tell him what she was going to do.

She just started wiping him down with the wet ones when she came in to work.

Even if he was asleep, she would start wiping him down.

I showed her how to bathe him in bed.

She continued to give him wipe downs with wet ones or wet washcloths without changing his T-shirt.

She was not able to get him out of bed for his appointments or in his wheelchair during the day.

On the days that he had an appointment. I got my husband dressed and out of bed to his wheelchair.

After his appointment(s), he would be sitting in his wheelchair and I had to get him back to bed.

It was as though I did not have anyone helping with his care.

She was consistent with confusing Amiaya and taking her to school.

James' pain pills were disappearing at a rapid rate. He received 240 pills from the VA. He was ordered to take 2 every 6 hours for pain. By the second week, he was down to 14 or so pills. He always ran out of pain pills before the next refill would come. He would go 2-4 days without pain medicine.

I developed a pain medication administration record. Angel was instructed to write down every time she administered pain medicine to my husband. She was instructed to administer 2 every six hours. I counted the pills left to ensure she counted appropriately to ensure his pills lasted.

James became more coherent and his pain was more manageable. Angel became more irritable and somewhat of an obstructionist.

She stayed in his room and would not give him privacy, even for me.

One day while I was once again showing her how to do a bed bath, she said,

"You can leave now. I have this."

I said, "I will leave when I am ready. This is *my* husband."

I should have said, "You can leave now, I've had enough of you."

I was stuck between a rock and a hard place. I needed help or someone at home with James until we finished the verification process.

We had offered the job to family members, those who used to visit often suddenly became unavailable to assist us, even with the offer of payment.

We were on our own.

I prayed that this was not affecting our baby.

Lord have mercy on us.

Angel became very territorial. And would not leave my husband's room, even when we told her that we needed private time.

She was cynical of how I was raising Amiaya and would not let her go near her dad to say good morning.

Amiaya told me, "Mommy, when I try to go in Daddy's room and say good morning to him, Miss Angel grabs me and holds me so that I cannot get to my Daddy."

"James is this true?"

"Yes. I tell her to let Amiaya go."

"Okay. Thanks for telling me."

She did whatever I ask her to do, even though she mumbled about it all the time.

She is always telling me, "You are so strong."

"Yes, I am. Is that a problem?"

Amiaya told me that Miss Angel says, "I'm sick of this job."

"Oh, really?"

"Yes, mommy and she is always talking when she leaves daddy's room and goes to the bathroom about how she is sick of this job."

"Okay. Baby, thank you for telling me."

"Mommy, are you going to fire Miss Angel?"

"I'm not sure at this time."

I was starting to feel really bad and did not know why my health was failing instead of improving since I had left my position at Walter Reed and Fort Belvoir. I thought that I was just over worked and exhausted.

Then one morning, it happened. I woke up with a fever of 102 degrees.

Thank God I had *an* Angel coming in.

Amiaya was home from school and I did not have to take her to school. I had taken that job from Angel.

I laid on the sofa in our bedroom all day just to get my health to a point that I could care for James when Angel left.

When she left, I would drag myself downstairs and give James his meds and water until I could no longer stand up. Then I would go lie on the ottoman in our living room and drink lots of water and take my blood pressure until I started feeling better. My heart rate was over 100 and Amiaya would not leave my side until she knew that I was feeling better.

When I started feeling better, I would get food together so that she and her daddy could eat.

Then I would lay down on the ottoman until I could get up again to go to bed.

This went on for 2 days.

Veterans Home Based Community Program

On the third day I knew that I needed to go to the doctor. I arranged for Angel to stay overnight and would have her take me to Fort Washington Emergency Room around 5:30 in the morning.

I knew from experience the Emergency Rooms were usually not busy on early Saturday mornings. From ten O'clock Friday night until four or five in the mornings were the busiest times.

If the moon was full, the Emergency Room was usually *Out of Control.* You did not know what would be walking through the door during those time.

The staff were usually winding down and getting ready for the change of shift at 5:30 in the morning.

I only spent two and one half hours in the Emergency Room. I had pneumonia. Wow!

I was shocked. This was my second time in 9 years with that diagnosis.

My baby made Miss Angel cook for me so that I could get back on my feet. According to Angel, Amiaya asked her to help her cook for her mommy and she started going into the refrigerator getting food out to cook.

"Mrs. Brown, I prepared a meal for you."

"Thank you, Angel."

"It was all your Baby Girl, Amiaya."

"Really?"

"Yeah. She said she wanted me to help her cook so that her mommy could get better. She started going to the refrigerator and getting food out so that I could cook. She even cut up the fruits and vegetables."

"Oh. My baby!!!"

I knew that my immune system was weakened from all of the colds and the stressful work environment that I had been in over the last four years. I seemed to have gotten one for every change of season. Even a daycare rash on my neck.

A rash that had the nerve to show up a few days before I ran into Montel Williams walking the halls of the old Walter Reed on Georgia Avenue in Washington, D.C.

I had been working on writing bonuses for the staff in the Trauma Department and needed to go up to the 5th floor to check on the progress of the paper work.

As I was walked down the hall, I saw a man walking with two other people.

It was if I knew this man personally.

I did know him.

I had watched him on television almost every day for 3 years.

It was Montel Williams of all people.

I stopped in the hallway after passing him and said, "Montel?"

He stopped and turned towards me and looked quizzically at me and said, "Yes?"

I think he might have thought that I was one of his old girlfriends he had left at the altar?????? Just saying.

I said, "May I shake your hand?"

"He conferred with the two people he was with. He must have seen all of that redness on my face and neck and thought that surely I must be contagious. I knew he had MS just like my husband. I knew that a hug was out of the question.

He agreed.

We shook hands.

I thanked him and he moved on.

That was the highlight of my day.

Wow! I actually met Montel Williams in person. He was a little shorter than I thought he would be.

I called my father and mother-in-law to tell them I had actually met Montel Williams.

Angel started to criticize my housekeeping skills.

Small items started breaking or scratches started appearing in the oddest places.

Her communication in our communication log became weird.

When I questioned her about clothes that I had found in my husband's laundry basket that smelled different with a strong odor. She told me that I "needed to speak to Mr. Brown, my husband". As if I did not know who my husband was.

She was fired on September 15, 2014, after ten months too long.

James and I were tired.

I needed help.

We took a month off before looking for someone else.

I advertised again on Care. Com.

We interviewed two candidates.

We gave one a trial.

This young man had just returned to the United States from Ghana. Before the Ebola outbreak.

We told him that we wanted to have him work for 4 hours so that we could make sure all was well.

I made Mrs. Carnathan aware of our intentions. She made us aware that we would have to pay him.

He reported on time.

He went in to talk to James and did his vital signs.

He came into the kitchen while Amiaya and I were eating breakfast and just stood there.

I asked him if he needed something. He just stood there and moved to the door to the deck.

He went back into the foyer and stood there looking up at the window.

He went back in the room with James.

On the way to school, I ask Amiaya how she likes him.

"Mommy I do not like him."

"Why don't you like him?"

"I don't know."

"Can he work with Daddy?"

"He can work with Daddy, but I still don't like him."

Out of the mouths of babes.

I returned home and went upstairs to get my desk space in order since I had to move my office to the bedroom.

I heard the doors opening and closing down stairs every 30 minutes or so.

I asked the young man if everything was okay.

He stood in the foyer and was just looking up at the window.

"Is everything okay?"

"Oh yes. I am just trying to see where the sun comes into the house the best."

"Really?"

"Yes. I love to be in the sunshine and outdoors as well."

"I noticed that you opened the curtains in the bathroom."

"Yes to let more light in."

I returned upstairs and a few minutes later, I headr a lot of walking and opening and closing of the piano bench in the Living Room.

It was almost time for him to leave.

I came downstairs to pay him for his time and tell him to keep working on the paperwork with Mrs. Carnathan.

"James, what do you think?"

"I think that he is okay."

"What was going on with all of the noise I heard?"

"He said he was looking for something?"

"Did you send him to look for something?"

"No. He just started rummaging through things in the Family Room."

"Oh really?"

"Okay."

"I will send him an e-mail and tell him that we are not in the program anymore and we will do it on our own."

"Are you sure?"

"Yeah. I am tired of people coming into our home and disrespecting it."

"Okay. I just want you and our daughter safe."

It was getting harder and harder to care for my husband. I really do need help. I decided to look at some of the people who responded to my previous ads. There were quite a few who had responded. I decided to call one particular person who seemed to have rehabilitation experience. She had even worked at National Rehabilitation Hospital in Washington, D.C.

"Hello. May I speak to Maria?"

"This is Maria."

"Maria. This is Cheryl Brown, I advertised for a Nursing Assistant on Care.com and you responded. Are you still interested?"

"Yes. I am."

"When would you be available to come in for an interview?"

"How does this week sound?"

"It sounds good. How does Thursday, 2 P.M. work for you?"

"Okay. That's good. I will see you then."

When Maria arrives. She is in the driveway for some time going through items in her van. She finally comes in and we greet her. She is escorted into the bedroom. James and I both interview her.

She interviews well.

We decide to hire her. She seems to have all of the necessary skills to work with James. She worked at National Rehabilitation Hospital in Washington, D.C.

She asks for an orientation.

I develop an orientation schedule.

Based on previous problems with employees wanting to become our family. I develop a contract for her to sign.

We negotiated a start date and time.

She renegotiated another start date and time.

I should have stopped there. I so needed the help and I wanted to go back to work.

She started work as scheduled and I spent four hours going through an orientation form to ensure she knows what to be done.

She became comfortable.

She told us that she had Gastric Bypass Surgery and is gaining some of her weight back.

I told her that I worked with Gastric Bypass patients at George Washington University Hospital.

I even gave her the Gastric Surgery magazines that I continued receiving in the mail. She read them and left them on the table. So much to adhering to the regime.

The microwave was beeping every 2 hours.

All of my teas disappeared within one week.

Food disappeared.

My dining room chairs started to fall apart.

"Maria, if you see something that needs to be repaired, can you let me know so that it can be fixed?"

The floor in the kitchen is scraped by the chairs every time she sits down or gets up. I hear a loud scraping noise while sitting upstairs at my desk working on our first book.

"Maria, do you think that you can stop scraping the chairs when you use them?"

I brought a ham for Thanksgiving.

"Oh Mrs. Brown, I just love those Honey Baked Hams."

"Well, this Ham is for Thanksgiving."

"I am leaving it in the refrigerator until then."

James asked for a Corned Beef Sandwich from the deli meat purchased from the Commissary. Maria was shown where the Deli Meat drawer was in the refrigerator.

James started eating his sandwich and said, "Cheryl, this is not Corned Beef. This is the Ham."

"Maria. Did you make a Corned Beef Sandwich or Honey Baked Ham sandwich for James?"

"Oh. Miss Cheryl, I made a Ham sandwich for Mr. Brown."

"Didn't I tell you that the Ham was for Thanksgiving?"

"Oh. I'm sorry."

"Please do not touch that Ham again."

James complained about his right side hurting.

He has a Baclofen Pump in his right side.

He tells me that on Tuesday, Maria tried to turn him on his right side and pushed him in the left side versus using his body to turn him.

I spent the next hour on the phone calling the National Rehabilitation Hospital and Georgetown Hospital staff. I wanted to make them aware of what had happened when Maria had turned James and that he was having excruciating pain on the right side where his Baclofen pump was seated.

On Thursday, I sent her with him to his Dentist's appointment.

The next week, I went with James for his appointment, the physician, and the staff members all talk to me about Maria's interaction with my husband while in the Dentist Office.

They said that she was "inattentive to Mr. Brown".

He almost fell on the floor when they were transferring him to the chair because they thought that she had him.

They voiced their concerns that she was not the one for my husband.

When I told Maria that she was going to be relieved of her duties via text message. She became very upset and hostile to me.

12/18/2015   4:38 A.M.

Maria. During my visit with James at the Dentist office, the Dentist and staff members voiced their concerns about your performance and my husband's safety. In light of this information and the incidents that have occurred over the last few days. I have no other choice than to let you go

The safety of my husband is very important and in good conscience, I cannot allow you to continue and am letting you go.

The hiring manual states that this is how it is supposed to be done by phone or e-mail.

I know that we need help, but I believe that my husband is too complex for you.

I do wish you the best of luck in your future endeavors.

12/18/2015   10:11 A.M.

I would just like to be able to address some things and speak on my behalf. I feel that is very unprofessional and not compassionate at all to send me a text regarding this matter. I would have liked to discuss this in person. I will be contacting the dental office to see how they felt Mr. Brown was not safe. There was no time during his visit that I was not attentive. I also made sure Mr. Brown was safe handled properly, and taken care of at all times. The dentist, dental assistant, & I had to work hard to (s) safely transport Mr. Brown from his wheelchair to the dental chair. Mr. Brown said that we did a good job. I am very compassionate and hardworking when trusted and allowed to do my job...Thus far I have done everything that you asked me to do. I am shocked and very saddened by this sudden change.

Maria

12/18/2015　　　　　　　　　　　　　　　　**11:37 A.M.**

Maria,

When I told you that proper notice would be given before letting you go, that was before the Dental Staff voiced their concerns regarding my husband's safety.

If I continued your employment and allowed you to continue to accompany him on Dental visits with the same things happening, I can be held liable.

Specifics; When transferring to the chair, they expected that you would be able to do so without help as I did on previous visits. James almost fell on the floor. When leaving, the seatbelt on his wheelchair were dragging caught in the wheels. The message was that you did not seem to know what you were doing.

When you hurt him the other day, I was willing to let that go, until my visit to the doctor's office.

Maryland is an, at will state.

I totally expected that you would be able to transfer/move my husband without me around.

I will not be held liable for injuries to my husband because I hired the wrong person. If you are unable to admit that my husband's care is too complex. I'm sorry.

Calling the Dentist's office will not resolve anything.
I've said all that needs to be said.
Please let it be.
Cheryl Brown

She was unable to let this situation be and sent another text:

"I am able to transfer hi. His seat belts were not dragging the ground because I buckled him in his seat. They had a hard time helping me transfer him. I will leave it alone. God knows and in the end He will have His say. Blessings to you and yours. Maria."

"Listen to what you just said. If you can transfer him, they should not have needed to help you. I didn't Please do not use God as a veiled threat because the God I serve is a fair and compassionate God. One who asks us to look in the heart of men; one who asks that we see things as they are.

I am sorry that you are hurt and upset. My family's safety is first and foremost and will be protected at all costs.

Blessings to you and your family.

It's over now."

She can't seem to cut it short. She continues to contact me regarding her time sheet. I instruct her to fax, e-mail or mail the document to me. She even sends a message via her husband's e-mail:

Dec 23 2014

Maria,
Good Morning.
    I re-checked my e-mail (in box and spam folders) and there is not an e-mail message with an attachment after December 14, 2014.
    I am not sure how or where you are sending your time sheet. My recommendations are this:

1. Send it by fax (301) 292-0346 after 9 A.M.
2. Send it by certified mail to my home address which you already have.
3. Send it to ASI and have Kimberly send it to me for signature or call me to verify days of work.

    If the above recommendations do not work, I am not sure what you need to do.
    I wish you the best in resolving this problem as I asked for your time sheet last Thursday morning.
    Just a follow-up on the incident with my husband:
    We had to call National Rehab Hospital because of how you turned my husband in bed by pushing him on his stomach versus turning him by his arms and legs. The pump moved in his abdomen and there was significant swelling around the Baclofen pump site. National Rehabilitation Hospital had us call Georgetown to speak to the Neurologist who inserted the Baclofen pump and advised us to continue to observe the insertion area because the edges of the pump were becoming visible. We have noticed that my husband is not getting enough

pain relief to his legs since that incident and are hoping that he does not have to have surgery to re-seat the pump. If it stops working, he could have Grand Mal seizures and die.

V/R
Cheryl Brown"

She failed to realize that she sent a message on her husband's e-mail. I responded back with the update on my husband's incident on his e-mail and he must have spoken to her because we heard no more from her.

Okay. We still needed the help.

What to do?

James wanted me to advertise on Care.com again.

I am so hesitant.

I advertised again.

Two nursing agencies responded to the ads.

I selected the one closest to our home, the one in Maryland.

Chapter 5

GREEDY UNHELPING HANDS

Okay.

Here we go again.

I called the agency contact person to see if they accepted the VA program and payment set up.

The coordinator assured me that we would be able to work something out.

I signed a contract to state that I would pay after the VA has been billed.

"Hi. My name is Cheryl Brown and I am calling to see if you can provide care for my husband. We have had a hard time getting qualified people to provide care."

"Oh, no worries, Cheryl, I am here to help the families in their times of need."

"Really. I have had a difficult time."

"What are some of the things that you have experienced, Cheryl?"

"Well, we have had things disappear, people ask for money, people who did not know how to give a bed bath or do basic nursing care, people who have destroyed our property, do you want me to go on?"

"Oh no. That's enough."

"Is Sunday a good time to come by? I think I have the perfect two people for you."

"Okay."

"On Sunday, I will have Mrs. Pansy meet me at your house and she can start Monday."

"I want to do a trial, next Monday, Tuesday, and Wednesday. James and I will discuss and make a decision. On Monday, I am going on a field trip with our daughter."

"Okay."

Monday, after the field trip, James said that things went well even though he did not let her do anything with him.

I watched him on the Security Camera and saw that the Nursing Assistant was with him most of the day except when she was getting something for him from the refrigerator or using the bathroom.

On that Wednesday afternoon, Mrs. Beverly, from the church called me to ask if I could come to her brother-in-law's funeral to be in attendance. I asked Mrs. Pansy if she can come in the next day and she agreed.

I contacted Mrs. Carnathan to make her aware that we had a person who came through an agency and the agency person said they could accept patients from this program.

Mrs. Carnathan sent the application and information for the accounting company. I gave the application, timesheets, and pay paperwork to the coordinator for the company.

"Latoya, I am giving you this paperwork because all of the employees who come to work fill it out and give it to the coordinator at the Department of Aging for Prince George's County."

"Okay, Cheryl, can you send me the paperwork?"

"Sure."

"I will look at it and let Pansy know what she needs to do."

A few days later, I contacted Latoya to let her know that the coordinator needs the application completed and the accounting office needs to have the payroll paperwork completed.

"Cheryl, I will tell Pansy she needs to get the paperwork to you so it can be sent in."

"Okay. You know that the money will go to Pansy's bank account?"

"Oh. Yeah."

"How do you plan to submit your invoice to get the additional seven dollars per hour that you are charging?"

"Oh. We will work that out."

"Do you think that you should still bill me for that additional amount?"

"I don't understand. How is the agency going to make their money?"

"Once that application is completed and submitted, Pansy no longer works for you, but the state of Maryland under the Veteran Community based program."

"She still belongs to the agency."

"She won't be working for your agency any more so the contract that I signed is no longer valid."

"You still owe me for last week."

"I don't see how I owe you when the Budget that you were emailed clearly states Pansy's start date of 1/07/2015. As of that date she no longer worked for you."

"No, Cheryl you owe me for that week."

"No I don't."

"Well, we can agree to disagree."

"Yes, but I do not owe you any more money."

"You said that you were going to pay half of the money that I paid Pansy for those 2 weeks."

"Pansy is going to get that pay. When she decides to leave, she will have 2 weeks in the bank."

"I am not going to pay you half when she will have the money banked up already."

"I will be by on Saturday so that we can sit down and sign new paperwork."

"You don't understand. Pansy no longer works for you. I am not signing any new paperwork with you."

"If Pansy does not want to come back to work she doesn't have to."

Email correspondence:

Latoya,

I wrote a check in the amount of $400.00 to Helping Hands and gave it to Mrs. Peterson to give to you for the remainder of what you paid her.

V/R
Cheryl Brown

———-Original Message———-
From: help <help@inhomeseniorNursing Assistantes.com>
To: Cheryl or James Brown <jcbrwnad@aol.com>
Sent: Sat, Jan 31, 2015 2:25 pm
Subject: RE: Fwd. Contract

    I understand. When we first spoke I remember you crying and in need have help with your husband. I started helping hands to help humanity not to cause any headaches. I will continue to pray for your husband. My heart is too pure to fight evil. I have never had issues with any of my staff leaving my agency and that will never happen. It will never happen because when you plant a dirty seed, you will get a dirty plant. I'm planting bless seed so I will have a bless plant. Now I understand why you will never have good people around to take care of your husband. Good will never stay around evil.

    I have learned in life never play dirty cause dirty never win and it's always a temporary win. I will continue to help god's people. This is my purpose and true calling in life. Helping people is my purpose in life and you are not strong enough to stop god's plan with me. All of this doesn't matter, what matter is your husband. I don't understand how you have time to be evil and be the devil' assistant. It is so sad you have time to play the devil's game. Your husband need all those time. You will never keep a good worker in your home for too long. I hope god clean your heart so good people can help your husband. Thanks and let god in your heart. Please do not call, text or email me or the agency.

Happy Connecting. Sent from my Sprint Samsung Galaxy S® 5 Sport

―――― Original message ――――

From: Cheryl or James Brown < jcbrwnad@aol.com>
Date: 01/31/2015 12:40 PM (GMT-05:00)
to: help@inhomeseniorNursing Assistantes.com
Cc:
Subject: Fwd. Contract

Latoya,

    I listened to the message you left on my answering service regarding "signing papers". I am not sure what "papers" you are referring to, but the contract is over and I want nothing else to do with your company.
    I've worked as a contract nurse, private duty nurse, assessment nurse (with an agency), program manager (government contracts), nurse manager (agency contracts) and once you notify the agency that you are no longer in need of their services, the contract ends.
    I am not going to sign any papers because I have terminated your services.

Have a great day.
Cheryl Brown

Greedy Unhelping Hands

———-Original Message———-

From: Cheryl or James Brown < jcbrwnad@aol.com>
to: help < help@inhomeseniorNursing Assistantes.com>
Sent: Fri, Jan 30, 2015 6:04 am
Subject: Re: Contract

Latoya,

Per our conversation, I stated that I would pay half of that amount because when she signed and submitted the application to PG Department of Aging during the week of January 12, 2015, the contract that I signed for you to provide an Nursing Assistant for me was made null and void. During our conversation, I also stated that you needed to subtract what I had already paid..

I have paid you since Mrs. Pansy came on board January 5, 2015 in the amount of 22.00 per hour for January 5, 6, and 8. The week of January 12 and January 19, 2015, you were still paid Assistant the additional 7.00 per hour for a total of 22.00 per hour.

When you answered my ad on Care.Com and I called you, I explained the program that my husband was enrolled in per the VA program that was administered through the Department of Aging. You stated that you would be able to bill the agency and then bill me after you received payment for the remainder due (third party billing).

I allowed you to work the process because you seemed to have it all under control. Normally when I hire someone, I make them aware that they do not receive payment for at least 3 weeks and the person understands that they will receive a full paycheck and will have be at least 2 weeks behind because of the pay system.

You conveyed inaccurate information to Mrs. Pansy and therefore, she expected to be paid as she had been paid through your agency.

Since I have paid you above and beyond the required amount for your agency, I also stated that that money could be used towards the amount that you required Mrs. Pansy to pay you.

I am discontinuing my contract with you, disenrollment from the program and go back to having the VA provide care through an agency.

I believe that a small claims court judge would agree with me.

I am not paying half of that amount because to date, you have collected $1,084 dollars from me.

You are not going to shake me down for additional money. I will see you in small claims court.

Cheryl Brown

———-Original Message———-

From: help < help@inhomeseniorNursing Assistantes.com>
To: Cheryl or James Brown < jcbrwnad@aol.com>
Sent: Thu, Jan 29, 2015 8:12 pm
Subject: Re: Contract

Per our phone conversation, you stated in the agreement between you and Ms. Peterson that you agreed to pay half of the $770 that was paid to Ms. Peterson. That half is due tomorrow 1/30/15 which is the agreement between Helping Hands and Ms. Peterson. The cleared check is attached.

Toya Baker
Client Relations Specialist
Phone 2402439500
www.inhomeseniorNursing Assistantes.com

———— Original message ————

From: Cheryl Or James Brown < jcbrwnad@aol.com>
Date:01/29/2015 5:11 PM (GMT-05:00)
To: help@inhomeseniorNursing Assistantes.com
Cc:
Subject: Re: Contract

Latoya,
 Please see attached.
 We will discuss in full tomorrow or Saturday.
 The terms of using an agency are not clearly spelled out in terms of who pays or how payment is delivered.

————Original Message————

From: help < help@inhomeseniorNursing Assistantes.com>
To: Cheryl Or James Brown < jcbrwnad@aol.com>
Sent: Thu, Jan 29, 2015 3:46 pm
Subject: RE: Contract

Strangers In My Home

Hi Cheryl, per our conversation earlier today. Can you please send over the documents you reviewed stating 3rd parties and 90 days? I would like to review them so we are both on the same page. Thanks

Happy Connecting. Sent from my Sprint Samsung Galaxy SÂ® 5 Sport

———— Original message ————

From: Cheryl Or James Brown < jcbrwnad@aol.com>
Date:01/24/2015 1:33 PM (GMT-05:00)
To: help@inhomeseniorNursing Assistantes.com
Cc:
Subject: Contract

Latoya,

I am still awaiting the contract from your company.

On Friday, I was assured by your husband that I would get it between 1–2 when he came to pick up the check.

We need to schedule a meeting to discuss the terms of the contract as soon as possible.

Thank you.
Cheryl Brown

On that Monday, James and I were anxious because we did not want to have any more confrontations with Latoya or her company.

Pansy came back on that Monday even though we did not expect her to. She stayed for two weeks.

She decided that her paycheck from the agency was not enough for her to come back to work for us even though she had 2 weeks in the bank.

My bathroom smelled of strong urine. I could not figure out why. I cleaned the floor, toilet, around the borders, sink, and all other items in the bathroom with bleach.

I even brought Lysol spray and Lysol cleaning solution to clean the commode and around it, since that seemed to be where the smell was coming from.

Finally, it hit me! Clean the wall behind the tank. Problem solved. Your guess is as good as mine.

Here we are again, out of a caregiver.

Here we are again, victims of extortion.

The person who does not have an advocate must really be suffering when it comes to getting someone reliable to help him/her.

My right hand and wrist have started getting weak. I believe I have Carpal Tunnel syndrome.

I brought a wrist splint and think that I will be okay until James gets back on his feet.

Pansy called after she got her second pay check with all of her hours. To wish us well on our visit to Kennedy Krieger and to let us know that she was thinking of us.

Think on, sister, think on.

I will take care of him by myself.

If I can no longer do it and the physical therapy does not work for him, I will have to place my husband in a nursing home with the help of the VA.

After finishing the program at Kennedy Krieger, I cared for James alone until May of that year. In May 2015, I called Cathy once again to ask for assistance to get my husband into the Charlotte Hall Veterans Home in Charlotte Hall, Maryland.

James has been there off and on for the last nine months. He did come home for a month after convincing me that he could do for himself. He continued to deteriorate and it was overwhelming caring for him so he unwillingly went back to Charlotte Hall.

Still no help from family. Not even his children.

We are truly on our own in this journey and it is indeed quite frightening.

I am still prayerful that he will "Dance with His Wife Again."

Chapter Six

HELPFUL HINTS FOR CARING FOR YOUR LOVED ONE

As you have read, it is very difficult to find and keep good help. I have worked as a Private Duty Nurse in many homes when I was a Licensed Practical Nurse. I never crossed the threshold of Patient-Client Relationship. There is a line one does not cross. As a caregiver, the person's interests are above your own

I never stole or asked my Clients for loans. I lived within my means and knew that if I was consistent, I would achieve my dreams of financial independence.

In an effort to identify individuals who were not capable of caring for my husband, I developed a Tip Sheet and forms to assist anyone going through this process to help with weeding out the incompetents.

I do hope that these tips and forms will assist you in your caregiving journey and you will not step into the traps that my husband and I did.

Tip #1

Activities of Daily Living take quite a bit of time. We have developed a system to make things work effectively by implementation of the following strategies for daily care.
1. Bathing is what takes the most time. During the winter months, bed baths are given at night. Sweating is not an issue this time of year because the heat is adjusted lower.
    a. When bathing, use a wash cloth to soap the skin with. When rinsing, use a different cloth to remove the soap from the skin
    b. Do not place the soaped washcloth in the water
        i. This keeps the water from building up soap residue
    c. I place a capful of Hydrogen Peroxide in the bath water as well
        i. It is an antibacterial and seems to work for us
2. Mouth Care is very important. If a loved one cannot brush his/her teeth, feel free to do it for them.
    a. It is very important to ensure dental visits are done twice a year for cleaning
    b. Repair of dental problems should be done immediately to prevent further problems
    c. Medications can make the mouth dry and a special toothpaste can be obtained from your dentist
    d. Teeth should be brushed at least two times per day
    e. Mouth wash should be used as well
3. Skin Care is very important.
    a. Oils and lotions can be used to moisturize the skin after bathing

Helpful Hints For Caring For Your Loved One

---

    b. It is important to clean the skin with warm soap and water after fluids spill on the skin

    c. Turning is very important to prevent pressure ulcers or bedsores from developing

    d. If there is not a special mattress on the bed you sleep in with a foam cushion, order one to put on the bed

    e. If a bed is delivered to the home from the medical supply company, remove the plastic covering

        i. The heat and moisture buildup can lead to skin breakdown

    f. Check the skin every day for breakdown

        i. If you notice the beginning of a pressure sore, ensure the area is cleaned with warm soap and water

        ii. If the skin breaks, use a protective barrier on it

        iii. We use a brand that is very thin and has an absorbable layer that helps the area heal quickly

        iv. We have also used shea butter on the area with relatively good success in helping the area to heal

4. Bladder Care is very important. If your loved one is incontinent or wants to prevent having accidents at home or in public.

    a. For women, use the disposable diapers, straight catheters

    b. Men can use the catheters or the external catheters

    c. Keep the genital area cleaned after each urination or catherizations

d. If external catheters are being used, clean the area daily and use a protective barrier wipe before placing the condom catheter on
   e. Clean the bags with an antiseptic solution, rinse the bag well and drain the solution out. Ensure there is a cover over the end of the tube on the bag when not in use
   f. Do not use the bags more than 3 days in a row
   g. Know the signs of urinary tract infection for your loved one:
      i. Strong smelling urine
      ii. Frequency of urination
      iii. Fever or elevated temperature
      iv. Burning on urination
      v. Cloudy urine in the bag or tubing
      vi. Lethargy
   h. Encourage 4 – 6 bottles of water every day
   i. Use Ellura to help prevent urinary tract infections
5. Bowel Care should be done every other day to prevent Automatic Dysreflexia in spinal cord injured or diseased patients.
   a. Use stool softeners, suppositories or enemas
   b. Eat lots of roughage
   c. Drink lots of water
6. Respiratory status is very important in your loved one when he or she does not move much. Buy an incentive spirometer from any medical supply store and have him or her use it if they are not on a home ventilator.

Helpful Hints For Caring For Your Loved One

    a. Use the incentive spirometer at least two times per day with an inhaler like albuterol

    b. This will help with preventing pneumonia which is a common problem with patients who have decreased mobility or who are bed ridden

7. Dietary needs change when you loved one is less independent. Appetite usually decreases and it becomes more difficult when there are dentition problems.

    a. Boost is a good source of nutrition

    b. Vitamins in conjunction with the physician's recommendations are important

    c. MS patients usually need vitamin D and calcium

    d. Increase water intake

8. Equipment to assist with the care of your loved one is very important. If your loved one is a veteran and is service-connected, equipment is not a huge deal. Some equipment items that may be helpful include the following:

    a. Accessible transportation can be obtained through the Veterans Administration with the appropriate paperwork

    b. Lifts and ramps for the home can be prescribed by the primary care physician by way of consult

        i. Vans

        ii. Lifts for vehicles

        iii. Lifts for the house

        iv. Ramps for the home

    c. Wheelchairs by way of consult if a Veteran

        i. Manual

ii. Electric
d. Scooters by way of consult if a Veteran
e. Chair lifts by way of a consult if a Veteran
f. Accessible bathroom and shower by way of the housing grant if certain percentage of service connection.
   i. Shower Chair
   ii. Railings on the walls to assist with getting up
g. Other supplies
   i. Bed Bags
   ii. Leg Bags
   iii. Blue Pads
   iv. Manpers (Male Diapers)
   v. Condom catheters
   vi. Holders for condom catheters
9. Exercise is very important for caregiver and loved one.
   a. If pain is a problem, get your healthcare provider involved to develop a plan of care to get relief of pain
10. Communication with your healthcare provider is key. Ensure you have all of the telephone numbers.
    a. Let the health care provider know if there are other physicians involved in the care of your loved one
    b. Keep all parties informed and share the information to ensure your loved one receives the most comprehensive care available
    c. Keep all vital signs recorded in a book
    d. Keep a log of medications with prescription numbers so that when ordering from the VA system, tracking of supplies and expiration dates are done appropriately

e. Make a log of treatment modalities that need to be done
f. Make an orientation check sheet for the caregiver to keep track of what is being done for your spouse
g. Make a communication log to use for the caregiver to document problems or concerns

TIP #2: CAREGIVERS

If you really need to have someone in the home, make sure you get past the first month with them in your home before leaving them with your loved one.

If irregular or unusual behavior is going to surface, it is usually during this time that it will happen.

Do not ignore the signs.

TIP #3: CONTRACT

Write a contract between you and the employee to ensure that you are on the same sheet of music.

The biggest problem I had was that every caregiver thought that he/she were on our level and that we had been friends for years.

I did not know any of those people and we were not going to be spending off duty time with them.

My contract included fraternization which is a military term. It was included to ensure the employee understood that he/she was just that an employee.

It takes time to become a part of the family.

TIP #4: DAILY TASKS

Create an orientation check sheet for the new employee and have them abide by it.

Having a communication log helped to ensure that information given to the employee was clear and if there were further problems, one could refer to the date the information was given.

Develop a daily treatment sheet. This includes all of the things that you want the employee to do with your loved one. It is very helpful to ensure turning or bed baths are done as appropriate.

TIP #5: ATTACHMENTS

See attachments at the end of this book that can be used to assist with creating an environment to help your family member receive the best care possible if you are faced with hiring outside help.

If you have a medical background, the hunt becomes much more difficult because as a trained healthcare professional, you know what to look for.

This manual was developed for the family member or significant other who is faced with making decisions in acquiring care for those they love most.

EPILOGUE

I have been a nurse almost as long as I am old. I started my nursing career after turning nineteen in 1978. My first job was as a Licensed Practical Nurse in the town of Nassawadox, Virginia at Northampton-Accomack Memorial Hospital.

The nursing program was subsidized by the State of Virginia because this was rural area and there was difficulty recruiting appropriate staff to work in the hospital. Physicians included. My first job was as a float nurse. When I reported to work on the evening shift, I had to go to the Nursing Supervisor's office and would be told where I would be working.

As a new nurse this was very scary. I never knew where I was going to be working. I worked in various positions as a Medication Nurse, Wound Care Nurse, Treatment Nurse, or Private Duty Nurse.

The Medication Nurse gave all of the scheduled and unscheduled medications for the patients on the unit. This job was one of the most rigorous. The goal was to ensure medication errors were not made. To make it through the shift without making an error was considered a major coup de grace.

We would wait in the nursing station until the next shift came on duty and counted narcotics. Only if this count was right, were we allowed to leave to go home. If the count was not correct, there was a whole process where security, nursing supervisor, and hospital administrator was notified.

I loved seeing the progression of a wound as it healed and always loved this particular aspect of my job. Most of our patients were burns or diabetic patients. Diabetes during that time seemed to be a foreign disease for all who acquired it. It was always so difficult for me to segment or compartmentalize that this was a disease which so adversely affected the African American population. Diabetes was one of the first equalizers that I had encountered.

After working for six months, I was sent to the Emergency Room and in my young mind, I thought that this was definitely an exit for me from the hospital. They were trying to get rid of me. I just knew it. Working in the Emergency Room afforded me the opportunity to start doing Private Duty Nursing.

The Hospital Administrator, Mrs. Arnold, knew of me from my ex-husband's employer. She approached me and asked if I would consider sitting with her Mother-in-law. I did not know what to do and was not certain if I would be able to stay up all night after working an evening shift. Mrs. Arnold assured me that it would be okay to sleep and only help when needed.

I must have done pretty well because I soon became the most requested person to work with people who needed a nurse to stay with them at night.

This type of work is what I gravitated to when I moved from the Eastern Shore of Virginia to Norfolk, Virginia.

Epilogue

Never once did I ever think that I could come into someone else's home and take over or take things that did not belong to me. I never once thought that I was on the same level as the family that I worked for. As an employee, I did not try to bring my whole family on and make it seem as if we had been friends for life.

Caregivers are supposed to be compassionate, kind, honest, trustworthy, loving, gentle, committed, and loyal and dedicated to the family they serve, but to the profession as well.

The experience that my husband and I have had over the last six years have been anything but extraordinary. We have had employees come into our homes who have lied, did not know their job, stole, hurt my husband and felt that they were not making enough money.

When I worked at Paralyzed Veterans of America and co-authored an article on "A Key to Independence", never did I ever expect to encounter the problems that I have in getting health care for my husband.

I've worked as a private duty nurse and never have I ever thought of treating family members the way that we have been treated.

I believe that most caregivers get a certificate to say that they are certified to take care of people in their homes as a means to get to the disabled person.

We installed cameras in our home to keep an eye on things. When I am away I can look in on James to make sure all is well with him with his Nursing Assistant.

When I started working as a nurse in the late1970's, it was an honorable profession and you had to pass the nun test of the directors running the program. A nurse in those days had to be honest, work hard and do the best for their patient.

There was a "prove yourself period". Once a new nurse or Nursing Assistant had passed this test, you were accepted into the group and worked continuously to prove yourself worthy of caring for those placed in your charge.

The nursing shortage has certainly watered down the types of people allowed to enter the profession. When I started working as a nurse, you had to love helping people because the money was not worth the type of work. Now the money is all people see when they apply for these programs.

So sad.

FORMS TO HELP WITH ACQUIRING THE RIGHT CAREGIVER

On the next few pages are documents that I created to assist me in acquiring the right caregiver. These documents assisted us in keeping the environment professional and helped us dismiss a caregiver who was not capable of taking care of my husband who is a complex patient.

ATTACHMENT #1: COMMUNICATION LOG

DATE	TIME	COMMUNICATION

ATTACHMENT # 2: ORIENTATION CHECKLIST

ORIENTATION CHECKLIST
FOR
JAMES A. BROWN, JR

Item	Expectation	Date Demonstrated	Date Completed	Initials	Comments
				Preceptor | Orientee	
1. Neurological	**Neurological** a. Identify level of alertness for client and document appropriately				

2. Respiratory	a. Identify Respiratory Problems and document appropriately
	   i. Shortness of breath
	   ii. Coughing
	   iii. Diminished breath sounds
	b. Understand use of Incentive Spirometer
	c. Understand use of inhaler				

3. Cardiovascular	a. Identify when vital signs are abnormal
	   i. BP
	   ii. Pulse
	   iii. Swelling				

4. Genito-urinary	a. Identify signs of UTI
	   i. Increased odor
	   ii. Burning with urination
	   iii. Fever
	   iv. Not feeling well
	   v. Locate supplies for changing condom catheter/bag				

5. Gastro Intestinal	a. Identify when client needs to eliminate
	   i. Listen to bowel sounds
	   ii. Understand bowel schedule
	   iii. Locate bowel supplies
	      i. Blue Pads
	      ii. Vaseline
	      iii. Suppositories
	      iv. Gloves
	      v. Enemas				

ORIENTATION CHECKLIST
FOR
JAMES A. BROWN, JR

Item	Expectation	Date Demonstrated	Date Completed	Initials	Comments
				Preceptor / Orientee	
6. Integumentary	a. Give Bed Bath and assist with Shower PRN b. Identify beginning stages of skin breakdown c. Identify supplies to apply to decubitus ulcer d. Understand importance of cleaning basin with Lysol wipes before storing on cabinet				

7. Musculoskeletal	a. Understand the diagnosis of Multiple Sclerosis
	   i. Read books from PVA
	b. Understand exercises to assist with rehabilitation process
	c. Understand how to use wheel chair
	   i. Turn on power
	   ii. Turn off power
	   iii. Move chair
	   iv. Charge chair
	   v. Manual Mode
	   vi. Seat belts				

8. Supplies	a. Know where supplies are located b. Understand how to order supplies				
9. Communication Log	a. Understand use of and need for communication log				
10. Care Manual	a. Understand the use of the Care Manual and dividers in the log				
11. Family Privacy	a. Understand role in the home is as a guest b. Understand that privacy and confidentiality is very important				

ORIENTATION CHECKLIST
FOR
JAMES A. BROWN, JR

Item	Expectation	Date Demonstrated	Date Completed	Initials	Comments
				Preceptor / Orientee	

12. Van	a. Understand how to use Van for travel to appointments
	   i. Understand how to use the key
	   ii. Understand how to turn on van
	   iii. Understand how to open ramp
	   iv. Understand how to close ramp
	   v. Understand how to lock wheel chair in van
	   vi. Understand how to unlock wheelchair				

13. Lift	a. Understand how to use lift to get to garage floor b. Understand how to use lift to get up to floor or house				
14. Lifeline	a. Understand how to use lifeline to call for emergencies				

15. Medication	a. Administer morning medications
	   i. Prepared by wife in med boxes on TV stand
	   ii. Give Percocet tabs (2) 1 – 2 times and write in composition book				

16. Vital Signs	a. Do vital signs daily and record in composition book
	   i. Understand normal blood pressure, pulse and temperature
	   ii. Report abnormal blood pressure, pulse and temperature				

17. Cooking/Cleaning	a. Understand that wife will do major cleaning and cook meals i. Report any spills to Client's wife b. Aide will prepare sandwiches/snacks for Client				

ATTACHMENT # 3: CONTRACT

Home Health Care

Contract

This contract has been written to establish the rules and expectations between the client James A. Brown, Jr and his caregiver, _____.

Upon employment at the home of James and Cheryl D. Brown, Mr. /Mrs. _____ agrees to support the client in the following endeavors:

1. Remain professional at all times. Both the client, caregiver and family members will maintain the highest level of professionalism at all times as evidenced by the following:
    a. Clients and Nursing Assistant will address each other appropriately at all times
    b. Clients and Nursing Assistant will not fraternize during or after duty hours.
        i. Fraternization is defined as attending events together, socializing in an environment that is not considered for business purposes.
    c. Communication written and oral will remain professional as evidenced by absence of profanity.
    d. Communication should be clear and concise so that there is no confusion between the clients and Nursing Assistant.
    e. Holidays and days off will be requested at least 1 week in advance in writing in communication log.

Forms To Help With Acquiring The Right Caregiver

    f. Sick calls will be done at least 2 hours prior to the start of work hours.

    g. Wearing of appropriate attire (scrub sets, jeans and scrub top or gym pants with appropriate top).

2. Respect the premises by doing the following:
    a. Do not wander around the house without purpose.
    b. Remain on the first floor unless instructed by one of the clients to upstairs or in the basement.
    c. Only vacuum/clean the Client's bedroom and bathroom.
    d. Wash dishes after meal preparation.
    e. Ask for items versus borrowing without permission.
    f. Inform Clients of problems identified:
        i. Shortage of supplies
        ii. Damage to equipment/household structure/appliances/van, etc.
3. Assist Client to gain independence by doing the following:
    a. Encourage to drink and feed self.
    b. Assist with passive range of motion exercises.
    c. Encourage to exercise on own
    d. Place items within reach (TV remote control, fan remote control, cell phone, water).

I _____ understand the above terms and agree to follow them while employed in the home of James and Cheryl Brown.

_____ Date: _____

_____ Date: _____

ATTACHMENT # 4: INTERVIEW QUESTIONS
INTERVIEW QUESTIONS

1. You are running late and when you arrive, the patient's wife has given him a bath and gotten him up in the chair. How would you handle this situation?
    a. The answer to this question will help you determine if the employee is a team player. If they are trying to hide their incompetency, they will not want anyone to help with the daily care.
    b. This also gives you an opportunity to evaluate your loved one's skin and look for breakdown.
        i. My husband was starting to get breakdown with the wipe-downs. His first since he had become less mobile. If I had not intervened when I did, he would have had a serious problem.
2. Mr. Brown has decided that he does not want to have anything done to him when you come in. How would you handle this situation?
    a. This will help you ascertain if the employee is willing to work with the patient and listen to the patient's desires.
        i. My husband is a late sleeper and one particular employee would come in at the appointed time which was usually at 5:30 since I was still working and just start doing things to my husband without listening to him.
        ii. He would tell her he did not want anything done to him, but she did not listen.
3. Are you proficient in giving a bed bath? Please describe how you would do that?

Forms To Help With Acquiring The Right Caregiver

    a. One employee was not proficient in doing bed baths at all. I now wonder if she had ever given anyone a bath at all.
4. Are you proficient in providing skin care and Foley care? Please describe how you would do so.
    a. This gives you an idea of how much exposure this employee has had to doing skin care and preserving the skin.
    b. If he/she is able to describe the frequency of turning, the importance of keeping the skin dry and clean and identifying when the skin is beginning to breakdown, they have had experience with complex patients.
5. Do you have a current driver's license? What state?
    a. If the employee does not have a driver's license for the state they are working in, background check is certainly recommended.
6. Do you know how to use a modified van to transport patients in?
    a. Most employees do not have this experience and have to be shown.
    b. If the employee professes to have this experience, have him or her show you on the spot.
7. Did you bring your credentials? License and CPR Card?
    a. For the VA Caregiver program, credentials are not needed because the program recommends use of family members or friends.
    b. Having CPR and a license is a big plus.
8. What salary are you asking for?
    a. Usually 15 – 20 dollars per hour is reasonable.

9. This position only pays 160 hours per month, for some months, there are more hours of work, and how would you handle not coming in when a month has more than 160 hours?
   a. We would work out something with the employee is he or she was okay with the VA program.
10. Do you have health insurance?
    a. Most employees working this plan did not have health insurance unless they were working another job or had a significant other or spouse with benefits.
11. What hours are you available to work?
    a. Most are open to the hours that you want them to come in.
    b. The person who keeps negotiating the terms of starting times is the one you have to realize will manipulate other situations.
12. What times of the year do need to have off?
    a. This helps you as well as the employee plan for time off.
13. Do you have questions for us?
    a. Questions should focus on:
       i. Physician appointments and frequency
       ii. Meals
       iii. Activities your loved one may enjoy or enjoyed before becoming ill
       iv. Family members or contact phone numbers
       v. Use of other equipment in the home
       vi. Are there areas of the home that I am not allowed in?
       vii. Cleaning
       viii. Trash
       ix. Telephone

QUESTIONS

1. What are your thoughts on the caregivers?
   a. The Liar
   b. Bait and Switch
   c. Unhelping Greedy Hands
2. What would you have done in each situation?
   a. The Liar
   b. Bait and Switch
   c. Unhelping Greedy Hands
3. Do you know people who have experienced similar situations?
4. How will you be able to help people going through similar situations?
5. How does this story impact the way you would deliver care to a Client in the home?
6. Do you think that people in the Health Care Profession should have an evaluation to ensure they are capable of caring for others?
7. If you agree with question 6, what strategies would you put in place?

REFERENCES

1. Bible, King James Version.
2. Key to Independence, PVA Magazine.